Leptin Resistance

Learn How To Take Charge of Your Leptin Hormone for Permanent Lifetime Weight Loss and Great Health

The Weight Loss Solution Series (Book #2)

By Sara Banks

Table Of Contents

CHECK OUT MY OTHER BOOKS

Introduction

I want to thank you and congratulate you for purchasing the book *"Leptin Resistance Defeated - Learn How To Take Charge of Your Leptin Hormone for Permanent Lifetime Weight Loss and Great Health"* This book is part of *The Weight Loss Solution Series* and contains proven steps and strategies to help you take charge of your leptin hormone once and for all.

Now that you want to lose weight where do you start? In the first book in the series,"Leptin Resistance Revealed" we had talked about how important it is to get your leptin problem under check if you want to lose weight. It is quite interesting that many people who want to go on a weight loss journey are always looking for the best diet to start on in order to achieve their weight loss goals without really making an effort to change their lifestyles and behavior that may be actually contributing to their weight gain. It is no wonder that most people who go on a diet usually end up regaining all the weight they lost within a year since they usually view a diet as a short-term solution. The other reason for this grim statistic is the hormonal part of our body. Our bodies usually want to maintain the status quo, meaning that if you take in less food, you provide lesser calories required for different activities and the body responds by being hungrier. This because our bodies do not want to change; that is why if you try to change things, your body responds by increasing your appetite hormones making you feel hungrier than before. What if I told you that the diet you want to start is not as important as being able to manage hormones well so that they can work for you and help you lose weight!

You may probably be wondering how hormones are important in enabling you achieve your weight loss goals. You need to understand that hormones control your entire body. Hormones affect growth and development, metabolism, reproduction, sexual function and mood. Therefore, this implies that if you want to lose weight, you need to ensure that your hormones work for you and not against you.

Leptin is one of those important hormones that you want to be on your side if you want to lose weight successfully. Leptin was discovered back in 1994 when researchers noticed that a mouse ate quite a lot but once they administered leptin, the mice lost weight. Leptin is simply a hormone that is produced by the adipocytes (the fat cells). It is some sort of way that the fat cells communicate with the brain about the amount of fat stores you have.

Leptin levels can be either too high or too low with each of these having negative effects on your weight loss goals. You need to have your leptin levels at a specific level, which is usually genetically set. At this level, the brain senses that the body has enough energy once leptin is released and thus enables you to start burning energy at a normal rate, eating normal quantities of food as well as engaging in energy consuming processes like puberty and growth.

However, if your leptin levels are low, especially when you start on a crash diet as explained earlier on, your body will not want to change and thus once you start losing weight (body fat), you will produce less leptin since your fat stores have decreased. You will end up being hungrier and have a greater appetite in an attempt to increase fat stores in order to restore your body to its initial position. This is why it is especially important to lose weight gradually to allow your body to adjust to the new condition rather than crash dieting.

You would then think that having high leptin levels is good as more leptin means that your brain can quickly notice when you have enough fat stores such that you do not need any more. However, it is not as easy as it seems. Having high leptin levels is not also good for your body. This is because once your leptin levels are high, your brain cells will start to become resistant to leptin meaning that you will need to eat more so that you can have more fat in order to produce enough leptin for your brain to notice that you have enough fat stores. Extremely high levels of leptin lead to a condition referred to as leptin resistance that you need to adequately deal with if you are to lose any weight.

In order to know how to handle the leptin problem effectively, there is need to understand what may cause leptin resistance. We will address this in the next chapter so that you can take the necessary steps to make the right changes if by any chance you are doing something that may be interfering with your leptin levels.

Leptin Resistance

There is no one single cause of leptin resistance but rather a combination of things that can cause Leptin resistance. We will look at the various things that can cause leptin resistance in order to know what could be causing the resistance in your case.

A Diet High In Sugars, Simple Carbohydrates And Fructose

Your diet plays a significant role in your developing leptin resistance. A diet high in simple carbohydrates, sugar and fructose is likely to lead to a drastic increase in your sugar levels once the carbohydrates are converted to glucose leading to release of insulin, which assists in the absorption of glucose in the body cells. Considering that simple carbohydrates and sugars are quite high in calories, the body will use what it needs with the excess glucose being stored as fat. As the amount of leptin is directly proportional to your fat deposits, the more fat you store, the more leptin you produce. As your cells are exposed to more leptin, you develop leptin resistance.

High Stress Levels

Stress can also be a contributing factor in making you develop leptin resistance. Usually when stressed, your body senses that it is as though you are in danger. This necessitates the release of cortisol, the stress hormone. Mild and periodic increase of cortisol is actually good as it provides a quick burst of energy for survival, reduces sensitivity to pain, increases immunity and heightens memory functions. However, it is the continued release of cortisol during stressful situations without allowing for relaxation and returning to normal that is bad for you as it leads to chronic stress. Higher and prolonged levels of cortisol in the bloodstream lead to suppressed thyroid function. The thyroid gland is an important part of the body as it produces important hormones that deal with metabolism. Metabolism is simply all processes that convert and use energy. This means that if your thyroid cannot perform as it should, you will end up not burning fat, as you need to. High cortisol levels are also associated with increased body fat especially around the abdominal part. This comes back to increased fat, which causes high levels of leptin to be produced.

High cortisol levels also causes an imbalance in the blood sugar levels like an increase in the blood sugar levels, which can easily lead to the storage of the excess glucose as fat leading to more fat and more leptin.

Overweight And Inflammation

Being overweight in itself will lead to leptin resistance since the more fat you have stored, the more leptin you will produce. This leads to insensitivity of your cells to leptin. Other than more fat cells causing extremely high levels of leptin being produced, being overweight or obese can cause inflammation. Normally as we gain weight, our bodies do not usually add more fat cells but instead, the fat cells expand and are filled with more fat. As these cells become stretched, they may leak the fats. Immune cells known as macrophages then come to clean the mess by releasing inflammatory chemicals in the fatty tissues. Our bodies may then respond by releasing anti-inflammatory chemicals, which then interfere with the functioning of leptin.

Crash Diets

Statistics indicate that most people who go on crash diets are likely to have leptin resistance. This is because most of these diets recommend that you almost eat nothing. A great reduction in your daily calorie intake can then cause your metabolism to be sluggish. Furthermore, you will be hungry all the time and your metabolism will decrease since the brain will be receiving the signal that you are almost starving; therefore, saving as much energy as possible. This is why it is always advisable to adopt a healthy lifestyle in order to lose weight steadily in the long haul.

Consuming Foods High In Lectin

Lectin has also been shown to cause leptin resistance. Lectin is a carbohydrate binding protein found in plants. It is usually found in high quantities in grains, legumes and dairy. Since lectins bind to carbohydrates, they are likely to do so in the small intestines. This may in turn damage the small intestines leading to a condition known as leaky gut. The lectins can then easily move from the gut into the blood due to damage to the small intestines. Lectins usually have a high affinity for leptons and thus will then attach to leptin receptors and interfere with the signal to the brain, which in turn leads to the need to consume more food in order to have enough fat to produce leptin. This ultimately leads to leptin resistance.

While it may be a little difficult not to eat all foods that have lectin, the key is to reduce consumption of foods high in lectin.

These are just a few of the common causes of leptin resistance. As indicated above, there is no one cause of leptin resistance but rather a combination of factors.

Now that you know what causes leptin resistance, how do you know that you are leptin resistant?

Common Symptoms Of Leptin Resistance

One of the most common symptoms among many people who have leptin resistance is insatiable hunger. You may just take what many may consider a satisfactory meal but still not feel satisfied. You may even find yourself eating too much until your stomach cannot take in any more food. You are also likely to crave sugary foods since dopamine is usually deficient. Leptin normally controls the levels of dopamine (feel good hormones); therefore, if leptin is not working, as it should, you are likely to want to find ways of releasing this feel good hormone. Comfort foods high in sugar and calories are quite good at releasing these feel good hormones. If you are leptin resistant, you usually become numb to sweet foods; thus, you will need to consume more of these sweet foods to get a rush of dopamine. You are also likely to be moody and irritable. This is usually because of a deficiency in the feel good hormone dopamine that is responsible for clarity.

Leptin resistance usually makes it very hard for you to be successful in losing weight. Therefore, if it seems as though you are not losing weight despite eating right and exercising, you could be having leptin resistance. In such situations, your brain could be actually thinking that you are starving and thus conserving as much energy as possible making it hard for you even to burn fat as you exercise. It could even make you feel hungrier, which means that you will probably feel the urge to eat more food in order to suppress the feeling.

Once you are done exercising and notice that you are taking an unusually long time to recover, you could be having a leptin problem. When you have leptin resistance, the body tries to conserve as much energy as possible since it presumes that you are starving when that is not the case. This leads to a situation whereby certain body processes do not function, as they should like lack of the production of testosterone, which is essential in recovery after exercising. In addition to this, exercising may be a grueling experience since you lack enough energy to exercise, as you should.

You may also have high blood pressure due to the increase in triglycerides due to increased fat, which then slow down the flow of blood, making the heart work harder in order to pump blood.

Having leptin resistance exposes you to a number of health risks as well as makes it close to impossible to lose weight and keep the weight off. What do you do now that you know you have leptin resistance? We will have a look at various methods that you can use in order to manage your leptin problem.

How To Overcome Leptin Resistance

Diet

What you eat is very important in determining whether you are dealing with the leptin resistance problem adequately or you are actually making things worse. This makes it important to know what not to eat and what you can eat.

Foods You Should Try To Avoid

Proteins and Fats: Milk, Ice cream, Fruit-flavored yogurt, Sunflower oil, safflower oil, margarines, hydrogenated fats, lard, corn oil, peanut oil, corned beef, peanuts, peanut butter, pinto beans, Lima beans, chickpeas.

Carbohydrates: Yams, White potatoes, pumpkin, muffins, packaged dry cereal, waffles, cakes, candy, cookies, chips, popcorn.

Fruits: It is paramount to reduce your intake of fruits high in fructose like banana, pineapple, grapes, honeydew and dried fruits.

You should also not take sweetened teas and energy drinks.

You would also need to stay away from brown sugar, honey, corn syrup, maple syrup and maple sugar.

Foods You Can Eat In Limited Quantities

Proteins and Fats: lean beef and pork, Fat-free plain yogurt, part skim milk, butter, coconut oil and canola oil.

Carbohydrates: low carb pasta and low carb tomato sauce.

Vegetables and fruits: parsnips, carrots, peas, strawberries, apples, apricots, blueberries, grapefruit, cherries, nectarine, peaches, kiwi, plums, raspberries, strawberries and pears.

Legumes: lentil and mung beans.

Foods You Should Take

Proteins and Fats: Fish and seafood like Tuna, Tilapia, shrimp, snapper, scallops, sardine, salmon, oyster, mahimahi, lobster, cod, crab, halibut, herring, perch. You can also take chicken breast and turkey with no skin. Some dairy products you can take include goat cheese, no-fat cottage cheese, no-fat cream cheese, no-fat ricotta cheese and feta cheese. You may also take tofu, both plain and herbal. You can also substitute some protein in your smoothies or meals by taking egg protein powder or whey protein powder.

Fruits and vegetables: The best fruits to take are avocado and olive since they are very low in sugar. Furthermore, avocado is very high in good fat. You can basically take most vegetables like asparagus, arugula, bell pepper, zucchini, watercress, turnip, broccoli, cauliflower, celery, cabbage, spinach, chives, cilantro, cucumber, eggplant, kale, lettuce, leeks, snow peas, seaweed, radishes, onions, parsley and rutabaga.

Carbohydrates: Low carb crackers, low carb tortillas, whole grain bread (if you have to) and manna from heaven bread.

You are also at liberty to use most of the spices like thyme, tarragon, tamari, cinnamon, cumin, curry powder, cayenne, black pepper, rosemary, paprika, oregano, fennel, crushed red pepper flakes, cardamom, capers, nutmeg, mustard, vinegar (red wine vinegar, umeboshi, balsamic) and dill weed.

You need to use oils like almond oil, avocado oil and olive oil.

You may take herbal tea, black tea and green tea.

As you have noticed from the food list above, your goal when on a leptin resistance diet is to reduce intake of high carbohydrate foods that have little fiber and increasing intake of carbohydrates that have more fiber. This is because carbohydrates like grains, cereals, breads, pastas and starchy vegetables usually increase your leptin levels tremendously. Furthermore, these foods are usually broken down into simple sugars that can be easily burned by the body. If your body is to choose between burning sugar and burning fat, it is more likely to burn sugar and thus the fat is not burned. Once it burns enough of the sugar for energy, the excess is stored as fat leading to more fat and thus more leptin produced. This is why it is especially important to reduce your intake of carbohydrates that can be broken down into sugar.

You would also want to increase your intake of good fats like those in fish and avocado while also increasing your protein intake and intake of carbohydrates high in fiber. While you would want to increase your protein intake since protein makes you full enabling you not to feel hungry too soon, you still do not want to overdo it, as too much protein is also not so good. You also notice that most of your protein will come from fish and seafood, which is good due to the high amounts of omega-3 fatty acids that are good in reducing inflammation.

Additionally, since we usually consume more of omega-6 fatty acids, you will also correct the imbalance when you take seafood and fish that is high in omega-3 fatty acids.

You would also need to increase your intake of good fat. Good fat is important as it enables your body to function. Furthermore, you actually need good fat in order to burn bad fat. Consumption of good fat will also lower the leptin levels to the required amounts enabling you to achieve leptin sensitivity over time.

You would also need to be aware of some important guidelines as you start on a leptin resistance diet

Do Not Eat Between Meals

I am sure that you have come across many different types of diets that encourage the consumption of five or even more meals distributed throughout the day. This may only be applicable if your leptin works well. However, if you have leptin resistance, it is advisable that you stick to three meals daily while having a break of five to six hours before the next meal. While this may seem hard, it is actually possible. Taking snacks may prove counterproductive since you will never know when to stop hence you will probably overeat on snacks.

Another scenario that may occur is that if you have three meals of a suitable size, your brain will be triggered to produce a certain amount of leptin especially since the size of the meal may not vary too much. However, if you eat a large meal for breakfast then a snack at ten or eleven, your body will not feel as satiated and thus, you are very much likely to eat more in order for the set amount of leptin to be released in order for you to feel satisfied.

Do Not Eat After Dinner

It is paramount that once you take your dinner, you do not eat anything later on. Eating after dinner usually increases the likelihood that the food you take will be stored as fat rather than used for various body activities. You should also ensure that you allow three hours after dinner before sleeping.

Eat A Healthy Breakfast High In Fats And Proteins

Breakfast being the first meal of the day needs to be a considerably heavy meal. You should concentrate on taking good fats and proteins that will keep you full for longer ensuring that you do not feel hungry. The good thing about good fats is that they make food tastier; therefore, taking good fats should not be a problem.

Exercise

The other important element in reverting leptin resistance is exercise. Once you adopt the leptin resistance diet, you would also need to start exercising. Exercise is known to alter energy balance regardless of diet composition. Exercise has also been known to activate leptin receptor-positive neurons in the hypothalamus in order to control body energy balance. Actually, exercising improves leptin's sensitivity in lowering food intake and body weight. Furthermore, we all know that exercising increases energy expenditure as well as lowering fat mass.

Once you start exercising, you can move from simple exercises to high-intensity exercises for short stints. These are usually advisable since they normally stimulate large secretions of the human growth hormone, which facilitate the body's fat-burning mechanisms as well as regulating leptin levels. A good kind of this type of exercise is high intensity interval training.

While exercise is important, you would want to start slow and build up to exercises that are more strenuous. This is because starting strenuous exercises when you are already leptin resistant will lead to exerting more pressure on the body, which leads to increased levels of cortisol and we know how that is not good. Increased cortisol levels are likely to lead to increased cravings and the need for overcompensation for the calories burned. While you can burn several hundred calories after spending some time on the treadmill doing some serious cardio, you are likely to feel hungrier increasing the chances of eating unhealthy food after the exercise session to overcompensate. Furthermore, you will also think that eating something tasting good (because you feel you deserve it) will not do much harm since you have spent quite some time at the gym. This could easily put you into a calorie surplus situation.

It would also be essential for you to know that over exercising especially doing too much cardiovascular exercise can have a negative impact on your thyroid function. T4 is usually the main hormone produced by the thyroid. T4 is usually converted to T3 in order to be used adequately for properly functioning metabolism. High levels of cortisol released during exercising impairs the body's ability to produce T4 hormone as well as suppressing the conversion of T4 to T3, which then leads to dysfunctional metabolism. Having a dysfunctional metabolism leads to decreased ability of the body to burn fat and lack adequate energy. Your inability to burn fat means that you are accumulating more fat and thus producing more leptin meaning that despite the fact that you exercise, you are making the leptin problem worse.

You should also know that over exercising normally brings the same hormonal effects that you have when you experience sleep deprivation, both of which make you leptin resistant. Your goal here is to overcome leptin resistance and not to make the condition worse.

So, what do I mean here when I talk about less strenuous exercises? Walking can be a great alternative. While walking may not provide the same calorie burning effects as cardiovascular exercises or running, it can be quite a healthier alternative for you. While you increase cortisol when running, you actually decrease cortisol when walking. Having lower cortisol levels is good for you, as you will not experience all the negative effects mentioned above of having high cortisol levels.

This means that you will be in a position to manage and control hunger and cravings enabling you eat less naturally. You also increase the presence of neurotransmitters like dopamine and serotonin that usually enhance your mood and general wellness.

You should try to walk as much as possible like a 30-60 minute walk for at least four days a week. Try replacing your cardio sessions with walking. You can also increase the fat loss by incorporating metabolic resistance training workouts into your routine as well as high intensity workouts that last around 20 minutes.

Supplements

While exercise and diet may be the best way to revert a leptin problem, supplements are also recommended. In most cases, adapting a leptin resistance diet enables you to get most nutrients. However, since you may not find certain foods easily, you can opt for supplementation of important nutrients you need in your body to combat leptin resistance. We will look at various substances that play a role in leptin reduction. Although the body manufactures some of these nutrients, you may still take them to ensure that you get maximum benefit from them. It is however important for you to follow the dosage as per the specific supplement to avoid overdose. You should also speak with your doctor to ensure that you do not mix certain supplements with medications, as this can be detrimental to your health.

Carnosine

Carnosine is manufactured in our bodies by combining amino acids histidine and alanine. The highest levels of carnosine are usually found in the brain and nervous system. In order for our bodies to burn fat, there is need for nerves to stimulate this. However, various reasons like aging and stress may lead to fat becoming less responsive to nerve stimulation. However, recent studies indicate that carnosine actually promotes the normal functioning of the nerves to stimulate the breakdown of fats through histamine receptors. Taking supplements is advisable to ensure optimal levels of Carnosine are in the body.

Pantethine

This is a dimeric form of pantothenic acid. Pantethine is usually an intermediate product in the production of Coenzyme A by the body. Pantethine can drastically improve your metabolism as it directly affects the production of Co-Enzyme A, which is an important energy broker molecule in your metabolism. Actually, it is used in over 60 metabolic pathways including the metabolism of cholesterol, carbohydrates and fats. Pantethine also helps in clearing toxins and boosting the adrenal gland function, which as we know is very important in your metabolism.

Pantethine is a derivative of vitamin B5, which has to undergo three enzymatic conversions for it to convert to CoA. However, pentethine only goes through one process. In addition, if you are leptin resistant, you are likely to have metabolic problems that impair the conversion of vitamin B5 further. Thus taking pantethine supplements is advisable.

Calcium

Calcium is very important in the body as it not only enables you have healthy bones but also assists in the indirect regulation of your weight. Calcium also regulates agouti-signaling peptide, which normally amplifies the production of leptin making it hard for your brain to respond to leptin. You would also not want to have too much agouti, which can lead to accumulation of excess abdominal fat, leading to high leptin levels. Therefore, you have to take calcium supplements to ensure such processes work well.

Acetyl Carnitine

This is one of the many forms of carnitine at work in our bodies. Carnitines usually carry specific fatty acids to the mitochondria to be burned as fuel. Normally, your body will produce its own carnitine with the kidney regulating the level of carnitine by getting rid of the excess. However, if your diet is low in carnitine, you may want to take some supplements. Since the body cannot absorb and metabolize fatty acids without acetyl carnitine, your metabolism will be affected if you do not have the adequate levels of carnitine. This makes it crucial for you to take acetyl carnitines supplements.

Vitamin D

It is quite interesting that although we can get vitamin D from the sun, over 50% of men in the United States suffer from a vitamin D deficiency despite it being a very important vitamin in fat loss. Did you know that having enough Vitamin D in your bloodstream will slow the accumulation of fat? However, if you have low vitamin D levels, levels of parathyroid hormone rise, which then turn your body into a fat miser making your body hoard fat instead of burning the fat. Studies done at Laval University and University of Minnesota indicate that having high levels of vitamin D reduces belly fat. Vitamin D is also a powerful inhibitor of the production of leptin from adipose tissue and is helpful in raising blood calcium levels, which is good, as you have seen the importance of calcium above.

CLA

Conjugated linoleic acid is made of several fatty acids isomers and is mostly found in dairy and meat. Adding CLA in your diet actually reduces body mass, which is important if you want to reduce fat. In addition, higher levels of CLA in the bloodstream also lead to reduction in leptin levels. CLA reduces body fat storage, enhances the synthesis of protein, reduce body fat as well as reduce leptin production.

Serotonin

This is a neurotransmitter involved in the transmission of nerve impulses. Serotonin is important in pain perception, mood regulation and gastrointestinal function like perception of hunger and satiety. Serotonin also has a powerful influence on our cravings especially for carbohydrates. This is why when we are depressed, we crave for sugars and starches in order to stimulate production of serotonin. However, if you take serotonin supplements, there will be adequate levels of serotonin in our bodies.

Omega-3 Oils

A diet low in omega-3 oils like DHA and high in omega-6 oils has been shown to cause a malfunction of the leptin receptor gene polymorphisms. However, high omega-3 oil levels with lower omega-6 oil levels are known to reduce this problem and ensure that the leptin receptors function, as they should. However, the leptin resistance diet is very effective in adjusting the omega-6 and omega-3 imbalance as it corrects this imbalance, as you will be taking more fish and seafood, which are very high in omega-3 oils. However, if you are still unable to get as much omega-3 into your diet, it would be advisable to take this supplement as it will ensure that the leptin receptors function normally. Furthermore, omega-3 oil like DHA oil is important especially for improving your metabolism making it an effective supplement.

Melatonin

This may also be referred to as the sleep hormone. Melatonin has been linked to producing a special kind of calorie burning fat. You can thus benefit by taking these supplements, as it may be of help in burning fat.

Zinc

This is a very important mineral that our body really needs. In addition to zinc boosting our immune system, this mineral also enables leptin to perform at its optimal level.

How to Take Supplements

It is important to note that supplements are not some magic pills that you can take and expect to lose weight when you have not adopted the appropriate leptin resistance diet. Supplements only work best when you eat well and exercise. In addition, you should also take supplements when you are unable to get some vitamins and minerals, as we do not want to increase your levels of a particular hormone or vitamin to extremely high levels such that you do not reap the benefits of taking the supplement.

You should also ensure that you take the supplements as per the required daily dosage. You would not want to overdo it and cause yourself more problems rather than make the situation better.

Alternative Treatment

Diet, exercise and of course supplements are crucial in managing leptin resistance. However, if you are looking for a less invasive way of managing leptin resistance and not having to take supplements, then you can also opt for various kinds of alternative treatments. We will look at some of these and how they play a role in managing leptin resistance.

Essential Oils

Essential oils are simply natural aromatic compounds normally found in the bark, seeds, roots, flowers, stems and other parts of plants. These oils are quite fragrant and usually give plants their distinctive smells. The different types of essential oils have been used for many years to treat various health conditions. We will have a look at the various kinds of essential oils that are useful in managing leptin resistance.

Grapefruit

As we had seen earlier on, when you have leptin resistance, you usually have cravings especially for simple sugars and high carbohydrate foods that are quite high in calories and eating such foods will only translate to the excess calories being stored as fat making the leptin problem even worse. However, using grapefruit essential oil can be quite useful in curbing cravings, as grapefruit has been known to be very effective in reducing cravings.

Peppermint

This essential oil is known to curb cravings ensuring that you do not overeat. Peppermint is also effective in suppressing your appetite and is especially great if you are leptin resistant since you never know when to stop eating.

Cinnamon

You are aware that having high blood glucose levels normally leads to any excess glucose being converted to fat for storage. Cinnamon essential oil is known to improve blood glucose levels ensuring that you do not have too much glucose and thus necessitate the storage of the excess as fat.

Ginger

Inflammation plays a key role in weight gain. Therefore, if you have to lose weight, you need to deal with inflammation. Ginger is highly anti-inflammatory, which aids in weight loss once the inflammation problem is dealt with.

Bergamot

As we have seen in previous chapters, stress increases cortisol levels, which then lead to more fat being stored. This means that reducing your stress levels is important in dealing with leptin resistance. Using bergamot essential oil is effective since it provides a calming effect and alleviates stress.

Lemon

When you have leptin resistance, you need to have your metabolism up and running in order to burn fat, as you should. Lemon essential oil contains a large amount of d-

Limonene, which is known for its metabolism boosting properties.

Lavender

Lavender is very effective for relaxing and calming. The scent rejuvenates, relaxes, soothes and slows you down when you feel tense and stressed. This ensures that your cortisol levels do not rise.

How to use Essential Oils

Essential oils can be used aromatically by diffusing in a diffuser or inhaling directly. You may also use these oils topically by applying them directly to the skin. It is usually advisable to dilute with a carrier oil like olive oil, coconut oil or any suitable carrier oil when you want to apply the essential oils on the skin. This is because the essential oil can cause irritation on the skin. Before using topically, ensure that you test on a small part of your skin and observe whether you will have any reaction. If you do not have any reaction, you are good to go.

While some essential oils may be taken internally, this is not usually recommended.

Massage therapy

Massage therapy has a number of health benefits that can aid in dealing with stress as well as weight loss. For instance, having a massage after an exercise is effective in enabling your muscles to recover and develop, which is extremely important if you want to achieve weight loss.

After a workout, your muscles usually need nutrients to recover from the strain. Since massage boosts circulation within your body, your muscles will receive the required amount of oxygen and other nutrients. When your muscles are able to recover from the exercise quickly, they are likely to undergo growth and development. Well-developed muscles are ideal since they help you lose weight by effectively burning calories even when at rest.

A massage is also effective in alleviating stress. We all know that stress is not good for you especially when you have leptin resistance as cortisol is usually released, which normally activates the storage of fat. Once you are not stressed, you will have normal cortisol levels ensuring that you are not storing more fat.

Reflexology

This is the application of optimal pressure on specific points and areas on hands, feet or ears. It is believed that certain reflex points correspond to different organs and systems and that pressing these areas has a beneficial effect on the organs and your general health. While this is debatable, reflexology has worked for many people; therefore, it is upon you to try what is best for you. If you want to lose weight, you can stimulate the thyroid area, which produces hormones that deal with metabolism to boost your metabolism. You can also stimulate the pineal gland located near the reflex area to the brain to suppress an overactive appetite.

A reflexologist may also target the midway down the left foot under the fourth toe. This area normally targets the spleen, which may also help in decreasing your appetite especially since if you have leptin resistance, you are likely to have a huge appetite and always crave for food.

Meditation

Did you know that meditation can help you lose weight gradually enabling you deal with your leptin resistance problem? Meditation is an old method of clearing the mind and calming your body. Most of the time, when it is mealtime, we simply start eating without calming down and enjoying the moment. When we do not concentrate during meal times, we are likely just to eat and even not notice when we are full until we can have no more. When you are leptin resistant and have a problem with your brain signaling that you are full, meditation can be very helpful. It may advisable to take a few deep breaths just before eating in order to allow your brain to be alert that it is mealtime and to concentrate on eating.

Breathing is important in bringing your mind to your food and enables you to taste the food and enjoy it. Doing this will actually help you enjoy the food and since you will be concentrating on what you are eating even when you do not fill full, you will know when to stop because you will notice that you have had quite a lot. Practicing this over time will enable you eat only what you need.

Meditation is also important for a clear foundation of healthier feeling and thinking. When you meditate, all clutter comes up; this includes negative body images, desires for certain unhealthy foods and emotions that may be attached to these foods. The more these surface, the more you can put these things in your mental recycle bin and start afresh. This is likely to enable you make healthier food choices even when you feel like you crave certain foods that will only make your leptin resistance problem worse.

Meditation therapy is also known to relive stress and create a sense of calmness. When you are calm, your cortisol levels will be normal; hence no excess storage of fat, which can lead to increased production of leptin.

Yoga

Yoga is quite effective in weight loss. Yoga is actually known to be suitable in fighting fat stores. Studies actually show that yoga can increase insulin sensitivity ensuring that your body burns foods for fuel rather than storing it as fat.

Doing some yoga exercises and postures is also effective in helping you calm and thus relieve stress. This is important, as you will not have elevated levels of cortisol, which can worsen your leptin resistance problem.

Yoga is also effective in suppressing appetite. Statistics indicate that more than 90% of people who practice yoga do not usually feel hungry afterwards. There are usually specific yoga poses that help your body control the hormones that normally make you feel hungry. This way, your appetite will be curbed and instead of having to control the hunger pangs, you will actually not feel hungry. Yoga is also effective in assisting the body to process food faster meaning that you get energy quickly. This helps with appetite suppression and weight loss.

Acupuncture

This is the stimulation of specific acupoints along the skin and body through methods like penetrating thin needles or application of heat or laser light. Acupuncture is quite similar to reflexology with the difference being the acupoints and the use of for instance needles.

Acupuncture is known to balance hormones. It also increases endorphins, which reduce cravings and thus reduce binge eating, which is common among those with leptin resistance. Use of acupuncture also reduces the levels of leptin restoring balance to your leptin levels. Did you know that you could also reduce stress by using acupuncture? As explained earlier on, being stressed increases release of cortisol and we know how that affects your system.

While all these alternative treatments are important in playing a role in weight loss through reducing cravings or your appetite for instance, you also need to eat well as these treatments work hand in hand with diet and exercise. You do not expect to eat crappy food and use one form of alternative treatment and expect to lose weight. Well, you might experience some change but for you to reap the maximum benefits of alternative treatment, there is need to eat well by adopting the leptin resistance diet.

A 5- Day Plan of resetting your leptin

So, how do you put into action what you have learned here. We will have a look at a five-day challenge that will help you reset your leptin.

Day 1

Diet

Breakfast

You can have deviled eggs and some vegetables like broccoli, spinach and asparagus. You may take a cup of coffee or tea with a little cream and a dash of stevia if need be.

Lunch

Chicken salad made of cooked skinless, boneless chicken, walnuts, avocado, lettuce and olives. Use olive oil, red wine vinegar, and Dijon mustard for the dressing.

Dinner

Rice with Grilled Shrimp

You may have some berries with low fat yogurt for dessert.

Exercise

You may exercise by walking for an hour. You can distribute this throughout the day. You do not necessarily have to walk for one hour continuously.

Supplements

You may take omega 3 supplements. Follow the prescription details to ensure maximum benefit from the supplements and to avoid overdosing.

You may use a diffuser for diffusing your favorite essential oils from the various essential oils for weight loss.

While snacks are not recommended, you can take some water or a handful of walnuts or almonds in case you feel really hungry. However, just eat a few to just subside the hunger.

Day 2

Diet

Breakfast

Turkey sausages with poached Eggs and one Granny Smith Apple. You may take a cup of coffee, black tea or herbal tea.

Lunch

Chicken Wrap: ½ pound cooked boneless, skinless chicken, dried tomatoes and chevre sprinkled with extra virgin olive oil wrapped with low-carb tortilla.

Dinner

Crab Salad with Avocado and Green Beans.

Exercise

You will still need to walk for one hour. As we have seen in the previous chapters, you do not want to strain your body as you can easily increase stress levels, which will probably work against you instead.

Supplements

You may take any other supplement depending on what you get from your meals, as supplements are suitable for providing vital nutrients to your body. You can also take the omega-3 oils.

Day 3

Breakfast

Mango Smoothie: blend one cup of cubed mango, ½ cup low fat yogurt, ½ cup water, 1 scoop whey protein powder and 1 nectarine.

Lunch

Turkey burger

Dinner

Broiled Scallops with rice

Exercise

Considering that you have taken a fruit smoothie and fruits are high in fructose, you will need to do slightly more intense workouts. A great exercise is high intensity interval training.

Supplements

As explained above, omega-3 fatty oil is one of the best kinds of supplement you can use. However, you can alternate between different supplements depending on what is lacking in your diet.

Alternative treatment

You may want to do a massage after the high intensity interval exercise in order to recover quickly.

Day 5

Breakfast

Zucchini Pancakes and a cup of coffee or tea with some cream.

Lunch

Greek Salad

Dinner

Chicken with cherry salsa

Dessert

Yogurt parfait: 1 cup low-fat plain yogurt, ¼ cup goji berries and ¼ cup raw granola (No sweetener).

Exercise

Do some yoga. Ensure that you get a good yoga instructor, as you do not want to hurt yourself during the yoga.

Conclusion

Leptin resistance is a problem faced by many people who are struggling to lose weight. This does not have to be you. With what you have learned in this book, you can take charge of your leptin problem and enhance your general body health. In the next book of this series, "Leptin Resistance Recipes" you will get a comprehensive list of delicious leptin approved recipes to help you in your journey towards curing leptin resistance.

Your next step is to check out a free preview of "Leptin Resistance Recipes – Delicious Leptin Diet Approved Recipes To Reboot Your Leptin Levels for Permanent Weight Loss Now" on the next page.

Thank you and good luck!

Sara Banks

Preview of "Leptin Resistance Recipes"

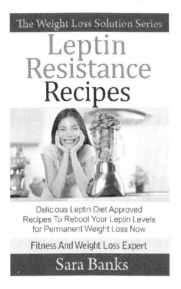

Leptin Resistance Diet

As explained earlier on, you need to be careful about what you eat when you discover you have a leptin problem. Your diet is very important as it enables you to address the problem slowly over time and as you do so, you learn how to eat more healthy foods. It is important that as you start on a leptin resistance diet, you know what to eat and what to avoid. We will have a look at some of these foods to enable you make better decisions.

What You Can Eat

Your diet should comprise of mostly vegetables and proteins with a little carbohydrates and fruit since most fruits are high in fructose (natural sugar). Below is a list of all the foods that you can eat:

Nuts: Almonds, Cashews, Macadamia, Hazelnuts, Pecans, Walnuts

Fish: Halibut, Herring, Tuna, Sardines, Cod, Crab, Lobster, Oysters, Salmon, Sardines, Scallops, Shrimp, Tilapia

Poultry: Chicken and Turkey with no skin

Dairy: Goat cheese, no-fat cottage cheese, no-fat ricotta cheese, no-fat cream cheese, feta cheese and Parmesan cheese

Vegetables: Zucchini, watercress, turnip, sprouts, spinach, snow peas, scallions, rutabaga, radishes, parsley, onions, mushroom, leeks, kale, lettuce, fennel, eggplant, cilantro, chives, chard, celery, cauliflower, cabbage, broccoli, bok choy, asparagus, arugula, bell peppers and artichoke hearts

Fruits: Apples, apricots, strawberries, blueberries, avocado, olives, nectarines, kiwi, grapefruit, cherries, peaches, pears, raspberries and plums

Ensure that you limit your intake of fruit owing to its high fructose levels.

Carbohydrates: Eat more of starchy vegetables and whole grain foods that are high in fiber like manna from heaven bread.

Fats and oils: Use avocado oil and olive oil mostly while using coconut oil, sesame oil and butter in limited quantities.

Use sweeteners like stevia in limited quantities.

You can use all spices.

You can have desserts like twice a week or even less times. You can instead opt for smoothies occasionally if you want something sweet but healthy.

What To Avoid Or At Least Reduce Intake

While it can be hard to list all the foods you should try to avoid or reduce their intake, your guide should be to focus more on eating whole foods, vegetables and fruits while reducing your intake of starchy foods, foods high in sugar as well as processed foods. While it is advisable to take fruit, try not to overdo the fruits, as some are quite high in fructose.

Dairy: Milk, Ice cream, Cheddar cheese, Swiss cheese

Legumes: Peanut butter, peanuts, chickpeas, lima beans, pinto beans

Vegetables: Yam, pumpkin

Snack foods: chips, cakes, energy bars, candy, cookies, breakfast bars

Sugar and Artificial sweeteners: maple syrup, corn syrup, fructose, honey

Fruits high in fructose like dried fruit, cantaloupe, muffins and waffles

All fried foods

Breakfast Recipes

Rosemary Eggs

Makes 2 Servings

Ingredients

2 eggs

½ teaspoon chopped fresh rosemary

3 tablespoons low-fat cream cheese

1 tablespoon fresh lemon juice

1 teaspoon avocado oil

1 teaspoon flax oil

1 ripe avocado

Pinch of cayenne

Salt to taste

2 slices of manna from heaven bread

Instructions

Mix the fresh rosemary, cheese, lemon juice, avocado oil, flax oil, salt and a pinch of cayenne on a bowl using a fork.

In a deep pan, add about two inches of water, bring to boil then simmer.

Crack the eggs one at a time in a cup and mix then slowly slip the egg mixture into the water as close to the surface as possible. Simmer the eggs for five minutes then remove using a slotted spoon and drain off using excess water.

You can then toast your bread. Cut the avocado into two then remove the seed and cut the meat with the skin on, then scoop the chopped avocado onto your toasted bread. Top the bread and avocado with the poached eggs and cheese mixture.

Hard-Boiled Eggs With Spinach

Makes 2 Servings

Ingredients

1 cup baby spinach

2 eggs

3 tablespoons flax oil

2 tablespoons sesame seeds

½ cup chopped fresh basil

1 teaspoon tamari

1 tablespoon flax seeds

Pinch of cinnamon

Instructions

For the dressing, mix the flax oil, sesame seeds, basil, tamari, flax seeds and cinnamon in a blender. Place the eggs in a saucepan, cover with cold water. Bring to boil and reduce the heat and simmer for 5 minutes.

Fill a saucepan 1/3 full with water, and bring to a boil then put the spinach and turn down to simmer for five minutes.

Cool the eggs in cold water peel and slice them. Drain your baby spinach and divide between two plates.

Arrange the sliced eggs on top of the spinach and drizzle with the dressing.....

Check Out My Other Books

Below you'll find some of my other books that are popular on Amazon and Kindle as well. You can visit my <u>author page</u> on Amazon to see other work done by me.

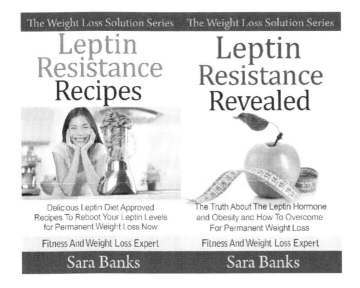

Printed in Great Britain
by Amazon.co.uk, Ltd.,
Marston Gate.